# HEALTH & WELLNESS

# HEALTH & WELLNESS

## SLOANE MONTGOMERY

# CONTENTS

# Introduction

The big question: what is health, anyway? Often melded with the idea of wellness, health is much more than simply eating right. It is a harmonious integration of all facets of a person's life, forming what can truly be described as a life well-lived. Health encompasses how one maintains and nurtures both the body and mind, aiming for that elusive feeling of fullness and well-being.

If you seek to understand the paths to maintaining a life of balance and stability, read on.

**Wellness**

Wellness is the pursuit of a healthy mind and body. It doesn't mean that every part of one's life is perfect; rather, it is about achieving balance amidst life's storms. Imagine life as a pie, with each slice representing different aspects that work together to create a whole. Creating a lifestyle that exemplifies wellness involves continual practice and a conscious effort to make choices that promote overall health.

It's about finding what works for you, practicing it until it feels right, and always seeking to challenge and expand your perception of health. A balanced life is one where no single area is neglected, ensuring the spirit is included and nurtured. True wellness is having the capacity to live fully, breathe deeply, hear clearly, laugh freely, feel intensely, see beautifully, and grow continually.

**Nutrition**

Instead of heavily restricting foods, focus on cultivating a deep awareness of the impact various foods have on your body. The core of this approach is balance – consuming nutrients and energy in alignment with your body's health goals. Understanding how different foods affect your energy levels, mood, and overall well-being is crucial in creating a sustainable and healthy diet. Eating a variety of foods in moderation ensures that your body receives the essential vitamins and minerals it needs to function optimally.

Incorporating a mix of fruits, vegetables, lean proteins, whole grains, and healthy fats into your meals can lead to a well-rounded diet that supports your health objectives. Paying attention to portion sizes and listening to your body's hunger and fullness cues can also help maintain a balanced approach to eating.

**Physical Activity**

Regular physical activity is another critical component of wellness. Engaging in activities that you enjoy, whether it's jogging, yoga, dancing, or strength training, can significantly contribute to your physical health. Exercise helps to strengthen the cardiovascular system, improve mental health, boost energy levels, and enhance overall mood.

Finding a form of physical activity that you enjoy makes it easier to incorporate into your daily routine. It's not about punishing yourself with strenuous workouts but rather finding joy in movement and the positive impact it has on your body and mind.

**Mental Health**

Mental health is just as important as physical health in achieving a balanced life. Practices such as mindfulness, meditation, and stress management techniques can help maintain mental well-being. Taking time for self-care, connecting with loved ones, and seeking professional support when needed are also vital components of mental health.

It's essential to recognize that mental health is an ongoing journey, and making small, consistent efforts can lead to significant improvements over time. Balancing work, personal life, and relaxation can help create a more harmonious lifestyle.

**Conclusion**

Health and wellness are not destinations but ongoing journeys. They involve making conscious choices to nurture both the body and mind, creating a harmonious and balanced life. By focusing on nutrition, physical activity, and mental health, you can cultivate a lifestyle that supports overall well-being and allows you to thrive amidst life's challenges.

# Chapter 1: Understanding Health and Wellness

## Learning Objectives

- Define health and wellness.
- Outline a definition of optimal wellness and well-being.
- Identify multiple facets of health and wellness.
- List several benefits of embracing a holistic view of health and wellness.
- Identify multiple areas of your own lifestyle that you wish to improve.
- Understand that no area listed in the DIMS/DOES sections of wellness is more important than another.
- Categorize lifestyle habits according to the impact they have on your health.
- Understand that making healthy lifestyle changes is a long-term process.
- Develop a process for setting baseline values for tracking a behavior change.

**Health and Wellness Are Holistic**

Our health and wellness result from more than just the physical interactions of tissues and cells. They encompass our connections with the community, employment, housing, recreational opportunities, educational access, spiritual growth, and personal safety. Managing our life issues or making changes in these areas can significantly enhance or undermine our well-being. Health and wellness are thus holistic concepts, integrating all aspects of life.

The Health Protection Model (HPM) provides a framework for understanding wellness. This course aims to teach students habits that balance the mental, physical, social, and spiritual aspects of their lives, promoting overall well-being. The concept of wellness is holistic, including social, emotional, spiritual, occupational, environmental, intellectual, and physical dimensions. The authors propose a Wellness Protection Model (WPM), similar to the HPM, which includes habits that improve quality of life and reduce stress across these dimensions.

**Wellness Key Terms**

- **Public health:** The study and efforts to improve the health of the public as a whole.
- **Holism:** The view that our life is defined by its holistic meaning—our life story—rather than a series of reducible physical events.
- **Health:** The physical and psychological state that is freely enjoyed by most of us; it is the presence of the positive in our life.
- **Wellness:** A quest to maximize health and quality of life by setting life goals appropriate to our energies, making life choices to meet our needs, and balancing our capabilities to achieve these goals.

- **Well-being:** Optimal health and quality of life possible with all seven dimensions of wellness (physical, emotional, intellectual, environmental, occupational, social, and spiritual) working together to support and reinforce each other.

## Definitions and Concepts

The Ottawa Charter for Health defined health and wellness as "the extent to which an individual or group is able to realize aspirations, satisfy needs, and change or cope with the environment. Health is a resource for everyday life, not the object of living; it is a positive concept emphasizing social and personal resources, as well as physical capacities." Promoting the health and wellness of students and student affairs professionals offers numerous opportunities and challenges. By focusing on hope, optimism, and resilience, research can positively affect mental health at institutions of all sizes.

The World Health Organization (WHO) defines health as a state of complete physical, mental, and social well-being, not merely the absence of disease or infirmity. Numerous terms and concepts related to health and wellness have emerged, including positive mental health, health promotion, wellness, health-related quality of life, and human flourishing. For some cultures, health and wellness encompass physical, mental, and spiritual dimensions.

Regardless of terminology, the goal is to not merely live symptom-free but to thrive. With government initiatives and updates to publications like Healthy People 2000 and 2010, we have entered an era where prevention is increasingly valued. Wellness, as a pursuit of a balanced, integrated, and satisfying life, is a worthy objective.

### Importance of Health and Wellness

In today's unpredictable world, health and wellness are crucial. Health is the ability to maintain homeostasis, recover from minor illnesses and accidents, and avoid severe health issues. An ideal body functions close to normal parameters and can effectively manage additional stress when required. Medical, psychological, and mental well-being are integral to overall health.

When these factors align, a person benefits not only from a happier life but also a greater sense of calm, improved self-esteem, and enhanced well-being. This includes diminished anxiety, reduced stress, and better performance in physical and mental activities. A healthy individual feels energetic, creative, and content. Maintaining a good diet, regular exercise, healthy habits, routine medical check-ups, and staying away from harmful substances are crucial for optimal well-being. Drinking plenty of water and including fibrous foods in your diet are also essential for maintaining peak health.

# Chapter 2: Physical Health

**W**elcome to Chapter 2 on Physical Health

This chapter dives directly into physical health, focusing primarily on the impact of a vegan diet. It examines three key areas under the Dimensions of Wellness program: Nutrition, Exercise, and Medical Self-Care.

As a philosophical note, I am not one to advocate for the "let's-get-our-sick-people-out-of-the-hospital-while-they-are-still-sick-and-just-give-them-some-drugs" approach. Nor do I subscribe to the "let's-permanently-cure-indicators-without-really-touching-the-actual-cause-before-he-sickens-again" mindset. Preventative care and holistic wellness are the main themes here. My goal as a nurse is to never practice acute care. It just may be possible to avoid such situations if we focus on keeping everyone around us healthy.

**Nutrition and Diet**

The term "eating habits" is only mentioned in the first subscale area. In the context of a wellness approach, "nutrition" and "diet" are frequently used terms. They are also prominent in strategies for improving wellness, which emphasize a responsible relationship with both oneself and others. The focus of our nutrition and diet subscale areas is to promote a wellness approach to physical disease and encourage the intentional use of this knowledge.

Nutrition and diet are not solely about being "healthy"; they are proactive steps toward preventing disease and illness. The importance of nutrition and diet cannot be overstated. Experts agree that the foundation for maintaining good health and preventing illness is established through proper nutrition. What you eat significantly impacts your well-being. Nutrition refers to the consumption of food that helps the body develop, prevent diseases, and maintain a sense of well-being. Both food and social support influence life and illness.

A key aspect of nutrition is understanding the best diet for weight loss. This includes projecting caloric intake, dietary claims, and physical activity requirements over the duration of therapy. Proper nutrition is essential throughout our lives to avoid health problems and maintain bodily integrity. The food we consume can significantly impact our body's ability to stay strong, regenerate tissue, ward off infections, and repair injuries. Conversely, poor nutrition can hinder the body's capacity to fight infections and recover from injuries.

Nutrients are crucial components of our food system, providing energy through six different classes: carbohydrates, proteins, lipids, vitamins, minerals, and water. For a human to thrive, they must consume food that contains all six macronutrients in the right proportions.

**Exercise and Fitness**

What is exercise? At its most fundamental level, exercise is motion. It is the movement of skeletal muscles that requires energy. This can be as simple as cleaning the house or working in the garden, or as structured as a scheduled game of tennis every week. However, exercise differs from physical activity because it typically has a specific purpose or objective. People often engage in regular physical activity to keep their bodies physically fit and strong, highlighting the strong connection between exercise and fitness.

Most physically active individuals exercise with some degree of regularity. They may lift weights, play basketball with an afternoon group, or jog daily. The good news is that anyone who is regularly active and willing to push a little harder can often become significantly stronger and faster. This improves muscle tone, posture, joint strength, and the ability to perform everyday tasks. Enhanced muscular fitness can improve balance, reducing the likelihood of falls and fractures, particularly in older adults.

Aerobic exercises offer the most significant benefits for the cardiovascular and respiratory systems. The long-term effects of regular aerobic workouts include increased life expectancy and a reduced risk of developing conditions such as heart disease and diabetes. Regular exercise of sufficient intensity and duration boosts the body's ability to store and use oxygen, a measure known as maximal oxygen consumption. This, in turn, increases the total energy the body can produce aerobically.

**Medical Self-Care**

The focus on medical self-care is about taking personal responsibility for your health. This means understanding your body, recognizing the signs of illness, and knowing when to seek medical attention. It also involves adhering to prescribed treatments and making lifestyle changes to prevent illness. Practicing good medical self-care can help reduce the need for acute medical care and improve overall well-being.

In conclusion, physical health is a cornerstone of overall wellness. By prioritizing nutrition, exercise, and medical self-care, we can create a balanced and healthy lifestyle that promotes long-term well-being. Through proactive and informed choices, we can prevent many health issues and enjoy a higher quality of life.

# Chapter 3: Mental Health

In this chapter, we shift our focus from the physical environment to the mental landscape. We explore how stress can evolve from a minor challenge into an overwhelming and confusing mess that affects our functionality. The solutions discussed here are aimed at non-relaxation, meditative techniques. However, we do not negate the importance of balanced physical well-being, which includes proper sleep and exercise programs. The benefits of physical activity and exercise on stress reduction and mental health are well-documented in kinesiology literature. For a comprehensive wellness plan, it is crucial to observe your physical well-being and apply some of those strategies to the complementary mental processes described in the following sections.

In particular, this chapter focuses on using your body to help support and assist your mind in achieving a calmer, more serene state. Techniques such as visualization, imagination, meditation, and creative practices are explained in terms of what they are, rather than how to do them. The goal is to provide you with an understanding of the intuitive inner workings and scientific marvels of your mind. By gaining this understanding, you will be better equipped to recreate these mental states through the specific examples and diverse creative outlets discussed in later chapters.

## Stress Management

The demands of academic life can be stressful, and managing multiple expectations can be burdensome. An essential aspect of mental wellness is our ability to effectively cope with stress. Stress is common and a natural response to challenging or difficult situations. However, when stress becomes overwhelming, it can lead to negative physical and mental health effects. It is important to understand that stress is not always something that can be controlled.

As a management strategy, behavioral and cognitive approaches have yielded useful techniques for making stress more manageable. The aim of these approaches is to reduce the negative emotional and physical responses that stress triggers. This is achieved primarily by altering the perceptions and interpretations that may arise in association with stress. While the stressor itself may remain unchanged, the way it is viewed or dealt with can be modified. Stress and negative mood often fuel each other, intensifying the negative emotional impact.

Research on stress-reducing methods, psycho-educational, and relaxation techniques reveals a growing body of evidence pointing to a range of successful strategies, many of which are presented in the following sections. Regular or intensive relaxation exercises are associated with psychological benefits, reduced stress, and improved physical health. Stress management techniques are built on a few conceptual assumptions. Stress management programs and treatments generally focus on two orientations: physiological and psychological. These procedures draw upon the premise that interventions are needed to mitigate the physical responses to stress. Evaluation of stress interventions indicates higher levels of effectiveness in treatments that concentrate on psychological aspects of the stress experience.

## Mindfulness and Meditation

Mindfulness is the act of observing and living in the present moment. It is beneficial for mental health, reduces stress, and has a calming effect. Furthermore, mindfulness meditation is proven to improve memory, attention, energy, positive emotions, and reduce stress. The positive benefits of mindfulness on well-being have been validated not only by scientific research but also by thousands of practitioners around the world for centuries.

Using mindfulness meditation to balance mental health and well-being requires a steady commitment to setting aside time and finding a quiet, comfortable place to relax. Adding relaxation music can enhance the experience. Here are some methods to practice mindfulness:

- **Feel Your Breath:** Close your mouth gently, close your eyes, and feel the air entering and leaving your body. Focus on your breath and notice the rhythm, speed, and depth of your breathing. Breathe in slowly and observe the rapid inhalation. If you find it difficult to focus on your breath or your mind is flooded with thoughts, relax and return to feeling your breath. If you encounter anxiety, acknowledge its presence and gently return your focus to your breath. Taking a deep breath and releasing it before finishing can also help. Meditation cushions can provide additional comfort and focus during your practice.

After practicing mindfulness meditation for a period, you may notice a reduction in anxiety, depression, and stress. You can also experience greater internal peace, love, and happiness.

# Chapter 4: Emotional Well-being

**B**uilding Resilience

Jim Delehaunty, founder of the Marin Teen Mental Health Collaborative, says, "It's important for all of us to get in touch with our emotional experience. We need to practice allowing ourselves to sit with any feeling we have and realize that it will pass and that we will survive... that's really critical." Resilience is essential for navigating life's challenges and stresses, and here are three strategies to help build it:

### Feeling All the Feelings

The reality is that we are inherently emotional beings. We all have thoughts and often emotional reactions to what we observe. Analyzing the swirling sea of emotions helps us put a label on what we are feeling, bringing clarity and understanding to our internal state. Emotions are not right or wrong but are communicators of information about our beliefs and passions. Expressing these emotions can open up the heart area, allow free flow of breath, and lead to positive emotional resolutions. Moving from feelings of hurt to a more reasonable state of acceptance or apathy sets us on a path to enduring peacefulness.

### Feel Free to Feel

Another strategy for building resilience is to accept our emotional nature and recognize that it is okay to be a feeling, passionate person without censoring our expressions. Whether it is an ex-boyfriend who hurt your feelings or frustration with the unrelenting hot weather, there is freedom in feeling frustrated, angry, hurt, or sad. Instead of suppressing these emotions, talk it out with someone you trust, cry, or express your frustration physically by stomping your foot. By not overly censoring yourself, you might find it easier to express love and joy as well.

### Building Resilience

Life can be incredibly challenging, yet individuals can adapt positively even in the face of difficulties. Resilient people manage to move on without being significantly affected by adverse situations, building rewarding lives. They demonstrate high levels of psychological energy and emotional well-being, and even amidst psychiatric and somatic illness, many continue to show adaptation and resilience. Resilience reflects a person's ability to cope with life's various challenges. Just as some people are more prone to depression and illness, others are adept at rising above adversity.

About half of resilience is attributed to "biological preparedness," while the other half comes from experience. To build resilience, one must first let go of rigid diagnoses, such as the belief that depression is solely caused by a "chemical imbalance" in the brain due to a genetic defect. This narrow view limits the range of solutions. Instead, redefining life as part of the common human experience allows for separation of the self from the illness, recognizing depression as a state of mind that can be influenced. The diagnosis of "depression" merely denotes a collection of unexplained symptoms. Finding a practical solution that works for the individual is crucial.

For example, regular physical exercise is shown to be as effective, if not more so, than certain antidepressant drugs. Engaging in activities like walking, even in the rain, and ensuring adequate sleep can significantly improve mental health. Dressing in a way that feels positive and empowering also contributes to better mental health, showcasing how practical steps can lead to a more positive and fulfilling life.

**Expressing Emotions**

Discovery Health reports that individuals who are able to express their emotions are more "emotionally fit." Emotional fitness involves understanding one's own emotions and empathizing with the feelings of others. Emotions play an integral role in our daily lives, affecting how we perceive the world, reason, communicate, and interact with others. When we are happy, we are more likely to see the good in those around us, help friends, and avoid confrontations. Conversely, when we are anxious or stressed, we might have a shorter fuse and fail to give others the benefit of the doubt.

Expressing emotions in a healthy way positively impacts overall emotional well-being. Many people feel better after a good cry or candidly discussing their worries, disappointments, or fears. Suppressing feelings can be debilitating, while turning to others for support can alleviate the stress of feeling alone. Sometimes, simply hearing yourself talk out loud can provide relief. Being listened to is inherently comforting, fulfilling our need for intimacy and security. Responding to the expressions of others also serves our own needs, fostering mutual understanding and connection.

By expressing our emotions, we reach out to others in a healthy way and connect better with ourselves, leading to improved emotional well-being and stronger relationships.

# Chapter 5: Social Connections

Strong relationships are incredibly rewarding, and numerous studies have shown that social connections can positively affect physical and emotional well-being. Regular social interaction has been linked to improved heart and brain health, particularly for adults over 50 years of age. Research indicates that seniors who are more socially active are less likely to develop dementia.

Having strong and well-established relationships with friends, family members, and community members provides a crucial support system during difficult times. Social relationships contribute significantly to emotional health and well-being. Staying close to others helps buffer life's stressors, providing emotional and physical protection. Involvement in social activities is associated with a greater sense of vitality and multiple indicators of psychological well-being. Forming a positive social network expands coping resources, helping to diffuse stressful situations as they occur. Participating in social activities can enhance your sense of joy, while also allowing you to receive and provide support.

Founded in 2020, Beyond Differences is a non-profit organization focused on ending social isolation in middle schools and raising awareness of its impacts. They offer strategies to help school administrators develop clubs and social activities. If your school does not offer a club that piques your interest, remember that you can always start one!

**Building Supportive Relationships**

You are worthy of compassion and understanding, just as those around you are. You don't have to face challenges alone. Reaching out for help or support does not signify weakness; it demonstrates strength. Building relationships and living a balanced life include expressing affection and love and actively listening to others.

**Elements of a Supportive Relationship:**

- **Enjoyment and Shared Interests:** Supportive relationships provide opportunities for shared time and interests, fostering a sense of ease and trust. Being able to break down without fear of criticism and expressing gratitude regardless of successes or failures are key components of such relationships.
- **Mutual Growth and Adaptation:** Relationships that draw you in are constantly improving and changing, allowing for personal growth and the development of new facets of your personality. Like a plane ride, relationships have their ups and downs, but the journey is made enjoyable through mutual respect and understanding.
- **Beneficial Partnerships:** Spending time together, smiling, enjoying, and nurturing one another in shared surroundings reinforces the importance of regular interaction. Maintaining control of beneficial or performance partnerships is essential for fostering time and individuality within the relationship.

**Community Engagement**

Emotional well-being is crucial for personal growth and flourishing. It is an integral part of overall health and wellness. Emotional well-being is often defined as the presence of positive emotions and moods, the absence of negative emotions, satisfaction with life, and the ability to function optimally. It encompasses the ability to rise above worry, demonstrate resilience, and include spiritual considerations. Emotional well-being is not just the absence of disease or disorder; it is the outcome of good mental and emotional health.

Emotional wellness involves the ability to feel one's emotions, listen to them, and use the information they convey. It means being attentive to thoughts and feelings and learning from the capacities and limitations they reveal. Emotional wellness includes feeling positive and enthusiastic about oneself and life, managing one's feelings and related behaviors, realistically assessing limitations, developing autonomy, and coping effectively with stress. It implies flexibility, balance, optimism, self-acceptance, and the ability to cope with feelings and limitations.

Strategies for enhancing emotional health and wellness in everyday life include a range of activities, strategies, and approaches for both workplaces and communities. Factors such as low socio-economic conditions, life stressors, lack of mutual trust and cooperation, and absence of supportive social networks can impact emotional well-being. Participation in community activities offers individual fulfillment and achievement while benefiting society as a whole.

# Chapter 6: Work-Life Balance

**I**ntroduction

In your quest for health and wellness, achieving a balance between work and life is crucial for success in both areas. These simple tips will help you on the work side.

**Effective Time Management**

The first strategy is to manage your time effectively. Several tools, such as time balancers and schedules, can help you improve your time allocation and management. The biggest task in effective time management is learning to set limits. This includes setting deadlines for meetings and phone calls, as well as designating a specific time when you will stop working for the day.

Time management is often described as the ability to do anything, but the reality is that there is not enough time to do everything. Balancing work, family obligations, social responsibilities, and personal commitments can be overwhelming. Regular exercise and healthy meals often get pushed to the bottom of the priority list. Stress, which is the accumulation of all the tasks and problems you have attempted to tackle throughout the week, can quickly make you sick.

To manage your time effectively, you need to examine your life to see what is important and what simply takes up time. You may find that you spend an hour or two each day mindlessly scrolling through social media or watching TV. By timing how long you spend on certain activities, you can identify areas where you can cut back. Additionally, assertiveness is key. Learning to say no when someone asks for your help can be difficult, but it is essential for maintaining your well-being. If you do not allow yourself time to relax and engage in activities of your choice, you will quickly become frustrated and burned out. Rescheduling your priorities to include time for relaxation and a healthier lifestyle will make you a more effective caregiver for others and improve your own well-being.

**Setting Boundaries**

The second strategy is to set boundaries between your work and personal lives. You need to learn when to work, when to focus, and what hours you operate best. You also need to recognize when it is time to stop working and focus on your personal life. Unfortunately, many people struggle with this balance. They see their work as an entirely separate entity from who they are, which can lead to several problems.

When you do not manage your work-life balance effectively, the stress you create in your personal life can begin to affect your job performance and the way your peers see you. Since stress is a common factor related to major health problems, including heart disease and high blood pressure, your health may also be impacted by ongoing tension. Ensuring that you have a balanced life between work and home can help guarantee your well-being and seize opportunities in life.

Setting limits or boundaries is a way to maintain internal and external balance to preserve your valuable resources of energy and integrity. This involves managing personal and professional stress and workload, identifying areas of life where the lines are blurred, and determining which aspects can be kept separate to provide a buffer when one area is particularly stressful.

Such areas include limiting personal time on the job, at home, and in the community, and finding time to be professional at work. Making good use of vacations, knowing the difference between appropriate self-disclosure and ethical secrets, and prioritizing the people in your private life are also crucial. The creation and maintenance of boundaries between personal and professional lives are fundamental to well-being, especially for professional caregivers.

While personal-professional life blurring and boundary violations are relatively common, the consequences can be more severe and costly in terms of long-term health and well-being for caregivers. Setting a limit on "giving" oneself to others, learning to say "no," asserting oneself in specific situations, valuing one's own needs and abilities, and having people in one's life who mirror back one's worth apart from one's profession are essential.

In conclusion, understanding and setting boundaries between work and personal lives, along with effective time management, are key strategies for achieving a healthy work-life balance. This balance ensures that you maintain your well-being and seize opportunities in life, contributing to overall health and wellness.

# Chapter 7: Sleep and Rest

L earning Objectives

1. **List and describe the three levels of sleep and identify the stage most crucial for physical restoration.**
2. **Explain the importance of sleep in mental well-being.**
3. **Propose strategies to ensure a restful night of deep sleep.**
4. **Identify the impact of sleep on athletic performance.**

## Introduction

In a world where the upper echelons are often rewarded for their abilities to work and compete for long hours, the significance of rest is becoming increasingly recognized. Researchers and coaches in the field of peak performance continue to explore the concept of rest in the lives of highly successful individuals. Napping, once stigmatized, is now embraced by many businesses that have created spaces for employees to rest and rejuvenate during the day. The mantra "meditation is the new medicine" has gained popularity, with coaches teaching clients how to meditate. Sleep, particularly in the competitive arenas of chess, business, and professional sports, remains a focal point of study for those interested in the habits of elite performers.

**The Importance of Sleep**

### The Three Levels of Sleep

Sleep is a complex biological process with multiple stages, each playing a crucial role in our health and well-being. The three primary levels of sleep are:

1. **Light Sleep (Stage 1 and Stage 2):** This is the initial stage of sleep where the body begins to relax. Brain waves slow down, and muscles start to unwind. Light sleep helps to transition the body into deeper sleep stages.
2. **Deep Sleep (Stage 3):** Also known as slow-wave sleep (SWS), this stage is critical for physical restoration. During deep sleep, the body repairs tissues, builds muscle, and strengthens the immune system. It is the stage where the body undergoes the most significant physical recovery.
3. **REM Sleep (Stage 4):** REM (Rapid Eye Movement) sleep is vital for mental and emotional restoration. It is the stage where dreaming occurs, and the brain processes emotions, consolidates memories, and clears out unnecessary information. REM sleep is crucial for cognitive functions and mental well-being.

### Sleep and Mental Well-being

The importance of sleep in mental well-being cannot be overstated. Adequate sleep improves mood, enhances cognitive performance, and increases resilience to stress. Sleep deprivation, on the other hand, can lead to irritability, decreased cognitive abilities, and an increased risk of mental health disorders such as anxiety and depression. Sleep helps to regulate emotions, making it easier to handle daily stressors and maintain a positive outlook on life.

### Strategies for a Restful Night

Ensuring a restful night of deep sleep involves adopting healthy sleep habits. Here are some strategies to help you achieve restorative sleep:

1. **Establish a Regular Sleep Schedule:** Going to bed and waking up at the same time every day helps regulate your body's internal clock, making it easier to fall asleep and wake up feeling refreshed.
2. **Create a Relaxing Bedtime Routine:** Engage in calming activities before bed, such as reading, taking a warm bath, or practicing gentle yoga. Avoid stimulating activities like using electronic devices or watching TV.
3. **Optimize Your Sleep Environment:** Make your bedroom conducive to sleep by keeping it cool, dark, and quiet. Invest in a comfortable mattress and pillows, and consider using blackout curtains or a white noise machine if necessary.
4. **Limit Caffeine and Alcohol Intake:** Consuming caffeine or alcohol close to bedtime can disrupt your sleep cycle. Aim to avoid these substances at least a few hours before bedtime.
5. **Exercise Regularly:** Regular physical activity can help you fall asleep faster and enjoy deeper sleep. However, avoid vigorous exercise close to bedtime as it may have the opposite effect.

**Impact of Sleep on Athletic Performance**

Sleep is a fundamental component of athletic performance. Adequate sleep enhances reaction times, reduces the risk of injury, and improves overall physical and mental performance. Athletes who prioritize sleep tend to perform better, recover faster, and experience fewer injuries. The Miller Laboratory for Researched Sleep has found that sleep prepares the mind for emergencies, supports maximal waking alertness, and bolsters a restful night filled with slow-wave activity.

For athletes who travel across time zones, mitigating the effects of sleep disruption is crucial. Strategies such as adjusting sleep schedules before travel, staying hydrated, and using sleep aids like eye masks and earplugs can help maintain a consistent sleep pattern and optimize performance.

In conclusion, understanding the importance of sleep and implementing strategies to ensure a restful night can significantly impact both physical and mental well-being. By prioritizing sleep, you can enhance overall health, improve cognitive function, and achieve peak performance in all areas of life.

# Chapter 8: Holistic Approaches to Wellness

This chapter will delve into holistic approaches to wellness, illuminating how integrative medicine marries complementary and alternative medical practices with traditional allopathic health care. We aim to expand our view from treating illness to fostering overall wellness, recognizing that an individual is a composite of mind, body, spirit, and emotions that respond to their environment.

**Integrative Medicine**

Integrative medicine not only seeks to alleviate physical symptoms but also strives to maximize an individual's vitality, health, and wellness. Guided by both evidence-based and traditional practices, it offers a multifaceted approach tailored to the needs of each patient. According to C. Prather, integrative medicine combines conventional and alternative treatments to offer the most appropriate care for each patient.

At the Office of Student Health and Wellness, a robust foundation in conventional medical practices is complemented by integrative strategies like meditation, acupuncture, therapeutic massage, and yoga. These practices aim to reduce stress, manage pain, and boost immune function. Office protocols developed by integrative physicians provide structured approaches to health and well-being, focusing on options that support overall health while minimizing side effects.

## Traditional Healing Practices

Traditional healing practices emphasize the importance of spirituality and emotional well-being, particularly within Native American communities. These practices, however, can be adapted for diverse cultural groups in public health contexts. Integrating traditional healing methods with biomedicine can be a significant aspect of achieving holistic health.

Throughout history, communities worldwide have relied on traditional healing practices and spiritual ceremonies. The significance of these practices varies across regions, religious affiliations, and cultural contexts. In the United States, indigenous healing practices have been marginalized due to colonialism, and African-based healing practices have similarly been overlooked. As biomedicine gains global acceptance, traditional practices face the threat of extinction.

## Ancient Wisdom and Modern Challenges

Ancient traditions of lifestyle wisdom continue to resonate despite the pervasive influence of Western lifestyles. Medical anthropologists like Carol Scholder, Joseph Campbell, and John Pilgrim have identified five key activities that facilitate healing: self-forgiveness and forgiveness of others, healing relationships, maintaining supportive networks, communicating about health issues, and finding meaning even in difficult times. These activities help people manage life-threatening illnesses better than conventional Western medicine alone.

Bodies with early-stage cancers, organ failures, and serious emotional disorders often respond more positively to holistic approaches than to Western-style surgeries and medications.

## Holistic Perspective on Wellness

A holistic approach to wellness involves recognizing the innate healing powers within individuals. It encourages the development of inner awareness to identify and transform destructive life patterns, creating support systems that help understand and address diseases. The focus is on achieving a balanced life through various strategies and fostering therapeutic relationships that prioritize the individual over specific techniques and interventions.

**The Role of Traditional Healers**

Different healers bring unique perspectives and methods to the table. The therapeutic relationship between healer and individual is emphasized over specific interventions. Traditional healing practices, deeply rooted in cultural significance, offer valuable insights and techniques for holistic well-being.

For additional reading on traditional healing from indigenous perspectives, resources like Onespiritprograms.org provide valuable insights into practices such as Hozhooji lifestyle changes in Navajo culture and the "Inipi decision."

By integrating these diverse approaches, we can explore what makes a healthy person and identify strategies for a balanced, holistic life.

# Chapter 9: Creating a Personalized Wellness Plan

Welcome to Chapter 9, where we will delve into what is undoubtedly the ultimate wellness tool: your personal wellness plan. This chapter will uncover the connections between the actions you took in the previous chapters and your journey toward improved health and happiness. You'll learn the significance of safeguarding your plan and ensuring it evolves to serve you best in the long term. Finally, we'll explore ways to create a doable plan and track your progress along the way.

**Why Your Plan Matters**

The "why" of your plan is crucial. In a perfect world, everyone would follow steps guaranteed to ward off hidden health risks, boost wellness, and foster a fulfilling life. If you struggle to remember to do this daily, this chapter offers a path to success through the development of a personalized plan. The most meaningful things you have learned will be translated into actions that can enhance your activities and life.

A wellness plan is more than just a list of tasks; it's a dynamic blueprint for your well-being. Do you need a plan to develop a more energizing workout routine designed to maximize the rewards of physical movement? The upcoming chapter will provide insights into various forms of physical activity, from running and swimming to other exercises to help you meet your improvement goals. Creating a stronger version of yourself now is key to aging slowly and building a powerful, versatile body. This book also focuses on nourishment specific to such goals and on becoming the best version of yourself.

## Setting Goals

Individual goals are as unique as the people setting them. Here are some questions to help you establish your personal wellness goals before we dive into examples:

- What does your dream state of living look like? How do you feel?
- What can you do, and how do you spend your time?
- How pleasant or joyful is your daily life?
- What are people saying about you, and what are you saying about yourself?

## Tips for Goal Setting:

- **Important:** Your goals must have real meaning to you. Determine what you want and believe is important. If the change is not significant to you or if you're making changes because someone else thinks it's best, sustaining the effort will be challenging. Assess the importance of this change in your life and its potential benefits to your well-being.
- **Clear:** Your goals should be well-defined and straightforward.
- **Manageable:** Set goals that are within your capabilities.

• **Controllable:** Ensure the goals are within your control, and you can influence their outcomes.

### Tracking Progress

Lifestyle changes generally occur over extended periods. Maintaining and monitoring these changes is vital. While some changes may bring immediate benefits, others will take time. Focus on sustainable lifestyle changes.

Though progress might be slow, the process itself is rewarding. By assessing changes, you can identify what works and make necessary adjustments. Many people find that creating a schedule facilitates a smoother transition. For instance, if you struggle to find time for meals, arrange for three meals and two snacks daily, ensuring you don't go more than nine hours without eating and eat every three hours. Keep healthy foods on hand to make this easier.

Remember, no two wellness journeys are the same. Acknowledge that this process will not be overnight.

### Case Study: Bariatric Surgery

Bariatric surgery can bring significant changes to an individual's life, improving relationships, work and social participation, health-related factors, and maintaining or continuing weight loss. Progress varies among individuals, and timelines depend on the surgery type. Setting small, measurable, and realistic targets helps achieve long-term success. Monitoring progress daily, weekly, or monthly shows your advancement toward a healthy lifestyle and achieving your goals.

### Continuous Improvement

When you reach a target, set the next one. Goals may evolve as circumstances and lifestyles change, necessitating periodic re-evaluation. Ultimately, the success of any wellness program lies in the value of changes in diet, physical activity, and behavioral modifications and the resulting improvements in health.

By embedding these principles into your personalized wellness plan, you can craft a sustainable path to better health and well-being.

# CHAPTER 11

# Chapter 10: Sustainability and Long-Term Wellness

Welcome to the final chapter of our journey towards holistic health: Designing Your Routine and the Concept of Sustainability. This chapter focuses on long-term strategies for transitioning from problems to solutions, with an emphasis on the sustainability of daily wellness practices. Since both getting well and staying well are crucial, crafting a wellness routine that you can envision practicing over the long haul is essential.

**The Concept of Sustainability**

The chapter opens with a thorough discussion on the concept of sustainability as it applies to daily wellness practices. Identifying ways to design a routine that not only addresses current health concerns but also supports long-term well-being is key. Sustainability means making choices today that will benefit your health tomorrow, anticipating challenges, and building confidence in your vision of enduring good health.

**Designing Your Routine for Long-Term Success**

This section is designed to help you shift your focus from problems and chronic disease to a mindset centered on good health. It encourages you to visualize your wellness future five, fifty, or even one hundred years from now. Sections will guide you through planning for the maintenance of good health you have or wish to achieve.

Being present in actions that promote wellness is just as important as recovering your health through medical interventions. The idea of wellness balancing is that neither problem-solving nor health maintenance is more critical; both sides of the scale are equally important. This section emphasizes the importance of focusing on both resolving compromised wellness and building and maintaining wellness momentum.

### Visualizing Your Wellness Future

To help you think about your operations to promote wellness now and in the future, consider the following:

- Envision your daily wellness routine.
- Identify potential challenges and plan solutions.
- Reflect on how sustainable your current practices are.

### Planning for Maintenance

Incorporate actions that promote wellness into your daily life. These actions are not just about recovering from health issues but also about maintaining and enhancing your well-being. Consider practices such as regular exercise, balanced nutrition, mindfulness, and stress management techniques.

### Wellness Balancing

The concept of wellness balancing teaches that fixing problems and maintaining good health are equally important. Addressing the issues that compromise your wellness is necessary, but so is implementing practices that help build and secure wellness-based momentum. This balance ensures a holistic approach to health, where both immediate concerns and long-term goals are managed effectively.

**Long-Term Wellness Choices**

Making informed long-term wellness choices today can signif-icantly impact your future health. Anticipate challenges you may face in maintaining your routine and develop strategies to overcome them. By doing so, you gain confidence in your ability to sustain good health over time.

**Conclusion**

In conclusion, Chapter 10 emphasizes the importance of design-ing a sustainable wellness routine. By focusing on both problem-solving and maintenance, you can create a balanced approach to health that supports long-term well-being. This holistic view ensures that your wellness journey is not just about overcoming current challenges but also about building a foundation for enduring good health.

# CHAPTER 12

# Conclusion

In this book, we have explored various strategies to approach health and wellness in a more balanced manner. We identified that current health promotion theories often rest on biased and false assumptions, such as an objective understanding of wellness, ideal states of health, and a strong commitment to individualism. These assumptions do not account for the diverse experiences and needs of different individuals.

We discussed three strands of thought that are usually marginalized within health and wellness research and practice, which have significant emotional, physical, and social implications. These include:

1. **People with Disabilities' Attitude Towards Exercise:** It's crucial to consider how people with disabilities view and engage with physical activity. Their experiences and perspectives can provide valuable insights into developing more inclusive wellness strategies.

2. **Scholarly Work Engaging with Pleasure and Satisfaction:** The importance of pleasure and satisfaction in promoting health and wellness is often overlooked. However,

enjoying life and finding pleasure in activities can have profound effects on overall well-being.

3. **Critical Psychological Work Focusing on Social Change:** This strand emphasizes the role of social change in health and wellness. Addressing broader societal issues can lead to more equitable health outcomes for all individuals.

While there is no easy answer to these problems, research and strategic thinking have convinced us that health and wellness should accommodate these perspectives as part of a balanced approach. Such an approach values differences, makes connections, and understands the intersections between various areas of life, such as leisure, work, and family.

Furthermore, we suggested that attention to emotions and endeavors, such as pleasure, satisfaction, friendship, citizenship, caring, and being cared for, is crucial on the path to health and wellness. These aspects are often marginalized but are vital for a holistic understanding of well-being.

A balanced approach engages with all aspects of a person's identity and is, therefore, more likely to have positive social outcomes. We proposed several dimensions of how an approach that incorporates our conclusions might work. For example, designing wellness programs that integrate emotional well-being, social connections, and inclusive physical activities can lead to more comprehensive health outcomes.

Finally, we acknowledged that while our approach has advantages, it also presents certain dangers. It is essential to continue researching and refining these strategies to avoid potential pitfalls and ensure that our approach remains effective and inclusive.

Overall, our conclusion emphasizes the importance of a holistic, inclusive, and balanced approach to health and wellness that values emotional well-being, social connections, and individual differences. Further research is needed to explore and address the complexities of this approach fully.